MW01168939

# EZ ECGs
## Booklet

Written by
Cindy Tait
RN, BS, CEN, CCRN

California Educational Update
Riverside, California

Publisher: David T. Culverwell
Executive Editor: Claire Merrick
Assistant Editor: Lisa Esposito
Project Manager: Peg Fagen

**Copyright © 1994 by Mosby-Year Book, Inc.**
A Mosby Lifeline imprint of Mosby-Year Book, Inc.

The author and publisher have made every attempt to
ensure the accuracy of the material contained in this
booklet. The author, publisher and their agents shall not
be held responsible for any adverse effects resulting
directly or indirectly from errors or omissions, or from
the reader's misunderstanding of the text.

All rights reserved. No part of this publication may be
reproduced, stored in a retrieval system, or transmitted,
in any form or by any means, electronic, mechanical,
photocopying, recording, or otherwise, without prior
written permission from the publisher.

Permission to photocopy or reproduce solely for internal
or personal use is permitted for libraries or other users
registered with the Copyright Clearance Center, provided
that the base fee of $4.00 per chapter plus $.10 per page
is paid directly to the Copyright Clearance Center, 27
Congress Street, Salem, MA 01970. This consent does
not extend to other kinds of copying, such as copying for
general distribution, for advertising or promotional pur-
poses, for creating new collected works, or for resale.

Printed in the United States of America

Mosby-Year Book, Inc.
11830 Westline Industrial Drive
St. Louis, Missouri 63146

Library of Congress Cataloging in Publication Data
ISBN 0-8151-0033-7

# PREFACE

ECG interpretation was once a specialty skill used only by physicians and nurses working with critically ill cardiac patients. Increasingly over the past two decades the ability to accurately interpret cardiac dysrhythmias has become a requirement of healthcare providers working in a variety of clinical settings. Routine ECG monitoring is now a standard of care for patients with cardiac-related problems. Additionally, cardiac monitoring is beneficial in the presence of any disease state or traumatic injury that may have an impact on the cardiovascular system.

The most recent standards established by the American Heart Association emphasize early recognition and treatment of life-threatening dysrhythmias. Accurate ECG interpretation is the first step in identifying these rhythms. The ultimate goal is to reduce the morbidity and mortality of greater numbers of people. Combined with good assessment skills, the ECG can provide useful information to help you choose a treatment plan for optimal patient outcome.

The *EZ ECGs* videotape and booklet were designed to assist the beginning student with the fundamentals of basic ECG interpretation. The *EZ ECGs* program can be used as a resource and review for the healthcare provider already interpreting ECGs within his or her practice.

The emphasis of this program is twofold. The first is to provide the student with the criteria for identifying rhythms originating from the sinus node. The second is to present the most commonly encountered serious and/or lethal dysrhythmias, i.e., rhythms that often require immediate action to obviate an adverse patient response. Therefore, not all ECG rhythms will be presented in this program. You may want to supplement your knowledge of ECG interpretation by consulting other references.

Case studies with rhythm strips are presented to provide you with scenarios similar to those you may encounter in your practice. Emphasis should always be placed on treating the patient as a whole, and not just treating the monitor.

Keep in mind that ECG interpretation requires memorizing specific criteria for each dysrhythmia. It is also a skill that requires frequent review and practice, as well as application in the clinical setting. Periodically review the criteria outlined in the booklet and test your skills using the scenarios in the videotape. The *EZ ECGs* program will help you build a solid foundation in the art and science of ECG interpretation.

Competence in ECG interpretation will be a significant asset and contribution to your clinical practice. We hope that you will find this program enjoyable, easy to understand and an enhancement to your practice. Good luck!

# Contents

# SECTION 1

## HOW TO USE THIS BOOKLET

*The cardiac conduction system*
*Etiologies of dysrhythmias*
*Interpretation tools*
*Important terminology*
*Standard ECG Abbreviations*

## HOW TO USE THIS BOOKLET

The goal of the *EZ ECGs* program is to provide you with specific criteria and interpretation techniques that will help you differentiate between normal, abnormal, and life-threatening ECG rhythms.

This booklet provides you with the fundamental information needed to evaluate each component of the ECG rhythm. You may want to review the cardiac conduction system, waveform criteria, and interpretation tools found in Section One of the booklet prior to watching the video. The video will then further reinforce the criteria that identify the sinus, atrial, junctional, and ventricular dysrhythmias.

The *EZ ECGs* booklet frequently elaborates on the information provided in the video. You may find it helpful to stop the video and review the information in the booklet.

It is important to have a good grasp of each concept before moving on to the next topic. Much of the frustration of learning to interpret ECGs can be eliminated by digesting the information in small segments.

A glossary of terms is provided on page 22. If a word used in the video is new to you, jot it down so you can look it up in the glossary. An understanding of the terminology used to describe the various aspects of ECG rhythms will help you better understand the concepts covered in the program. Also, a working knowledge of ECG terminology will improve your ability to accurately document your patients' dysrhythmias and to discuss your findings with other members of the healthcare team.

Section Two presents the criteria for identifying rhythms that originate from the sinus node. It is important to be able to identify the normally conducted ECG rhythms. Once you are able to recognize the sinus rhythms, you will find it easier to identify many of the abnormal ECG patterns that originate from other areas within the conduction system.

Section Three outlines the criteria for dysrhythmias that originate outside of the sinus node. These dysrhythmias are divided into sections based on their anatomical origin in the heart and are placed into the categories of atrial, junctional, and ventricular. Many of the dysrhythmias are further categorized as either ectopic, escape, or blocked rhythms.

Section Four is to be used in conjunction with the scenarios presented on the videotape. Open the booklet to this section as the scenarios are given so that you have a static copy of the rhythm and all of the vital information in front of you. You may want to stop the tape so that you can take your time. The exact same strip is shown in the booklet so that you can evaluate the waveforms more closely and measure the intervals. Also, by using both the video rhythms and hard copy strips, you will become more versatile in your ability to interpret ECGs in a variety of patient care settings.

Section Five includes a comprehensive quiz to test your ECG knowledge and interpretation skills.

Since you may not encounter all of the rhythms presented in this program on a regular basis, occasional review will help you maintain and continue to build strong ECG skills. Keep this handy *EZ ECGs* booklet with you as a quick reference guide as you gain confidence and competence in your ECG skills.

## The Cardiac Conduction System

The metabolic processes of the human body depend upon the ability of the heart to pump oxygenated blood and nutrients to the tissues. Movement of blood through the cardiovascular system is accomplished when the heart muscles respond to electrical stimulation by contracting. Blood enters the right side of the heart via the vena cava and is pumped into the pulmonary circulation. The left side of the heart receives the oxygenated blood from the pulmonary system and pumps it to the organs and tissues via the systemic circulation (see Fig. 1-1).

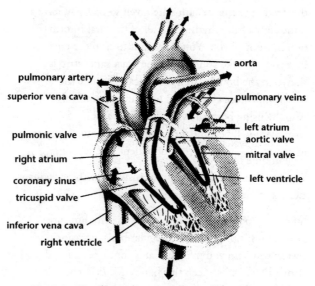

*Fig. 1-1. Circulation through the heart. (From Huszar RJ: Basic dysrhythmias: interpretation and management, 2e, St. Louis, 1994, Mosby.)*

The heart contains two types of specialized cells:

1. **Working cells** - the working cells of the heart are the muscular portions of the atria and ventricles. When stimulated by an electrical impulse, the working cells contract and pump blood to the lungs and tissues of the body. This process is the result of cellular depolarization, which occurs when electrolytes travel across the cell membrane causing a shortening of the muscle fiber. Repolarization occurs when the electrolytes move back across the cell membrane rendering the cell ready for the next electrical impulse. The status of the working

cells can be evaluated by assessing the patient's hemodynamic status, i.e., pulse, blood pressure, skin signs,
urine output, and level of consciousness.

**2. Conduction cells** - electrical impulses are transmitted
through the heart via specialized conduction cells.
During a normal cardiac cycle electrical impulses begin
in the sinoatrial (SA) node and are relayed through the
conduction system. The electrical impulses terminate in
the Purkinje fibers implanted within the myocardium.
The working cells respond to the stimulation by contracting. The frequency of these impulses determine the
heart rate. The heart rate is primarily influenced by the
autonomic nervous system's response to the demands of
the body for oxygenated blood. The status of the conduction system can be evaluated by interpreting the various components of the ECG tracing.

The cardiac conduction system consists of the **sinoatrial
(SA) node**, the **interatrial and internodal conduction
tracts**, the **atrioventricular (AV) node**, the **bundle of
His** (the region of the AV node and the Bundle of His
is called the AV junction), the left and right **bundle
branches**, and the **Purkinje fibers**, as seen in Fig. 1-2.
Each node or region is capable of acting as the pacemaker of the heart. Should the SA node fail to act as the
primary pacemaker, another site within the conduction
system often takes over. This is called an escape pacemaker. As a general rule, the further down the conduction system, the slower the rate of the escape rhythm.
The inherent rate for each site is indicated in Fig. 1-3.

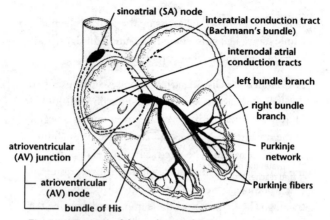

*Fig. 1-2. Anatomy of the cardiac conduction system. (From Huszar RJ: Basic dysrhythmias: interpretation and management, 2e, St. Louis, 1994, Mosby.)*

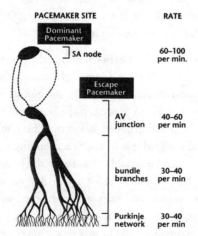

*Fig. 1-3. Dominant and escape pacemakers. (From Huszar RJ: Basic dysrhythmias: interpretation and management, 2e, St. Louis, 1994, Mosby.)*

Each ECG waveform represents electrical activity within a specific area of the heart. Knowing which waveform correlates with each area of the cardiac conduction system will help you to determine normal from abnormal conduction.

As seen in Fig. 1-4, a complete cardiac cycle has five identifiable waveforms. These electrical impulse patterns are labeled the **P, Q, R, S,** and **T** waves. In the

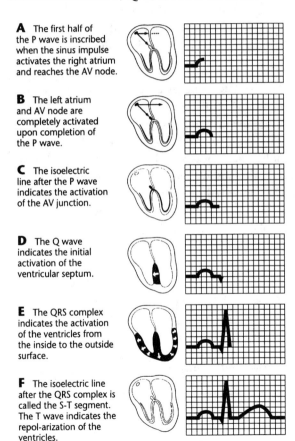

**A** The first half of the P wave is inscribed when the sinus impulse activates the right atrium and reaches the AV node.

**B** The left atrium and AV node are completely activated upon completion of the P wave.

**C** The isoelectric line after the P wave indicates the activation of the AV junction.

**D** The Q wave indicates the initial activation of the ventricular septum.

**E** The QRS complex indicates the activation of the ventricles from the inside to the outside surface.

**F** The isoelectric line after the QRS complex is called the S-T segment. The T wave indicates the repol-arization of the ventricles.

*Fig. 1-4. Cardiac activation and ECG (From Conover MS: Understanding electrocardiography: arrythmias and the 12-lead ECG, St. Louis, 1992, Mosby.)*

commonly used perspective of lead II, normal criteria for each waveform can be defined as:

*P wave* - represents depolarization of both atria. A normal **P wave** corresponds with the contraction of the atria and movement of blood into the ventricles. In lead II, a normal **P wave** will be upright and rounded. The **P wave** is identified as the first deviation from the baseline at the beginning of the cardiac cycle.

*QRS complex* - represents depolarization of the ventricles. The **QRS complex** corresponds with the closure of the atrioventricular (AV) valves which create the "lubb" sound during ausculation of the heart (see Fig. 1-5). The **Q wave** is the first negative deflection in the cardiac cycle not preceded by an **R wave**. The **R wave** is the first positive deflection in the **QRS complex**. The **S wave** is the negative deflection that follows the **R wave**. The **QRS complex** is also referred to as the systolic, or contraction phase of the cardiac cycle.

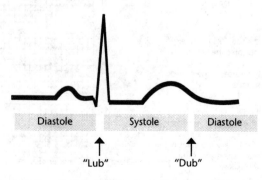

*Fig. 1-5. Systolic and diastolic phases of cardiac conduction.*

*T wave* - represents the *repolarization* of the ventricles. The end of the T wave indicates closure of the pulmonic and aortic (semilunar) valves which create the "dubb" sound (see Fig. 1-5). The **T wave** is the first deviation after the brief segment following the S wave. A normal **T wave** will be upright and rounded and should not be notched or peaked. It is during the **T wave** that the ventricles are returning to an electrically ready state to receive the next impulse. The **T wave** is also referred to as the diastolic, or resting phase of the cardiac cycle.

In addition to evaluating each waveform of the cardiac cycle, important information can be gathered by measuring the intervals between the waveforms. The illustration in (Fig. 1-6) shows the beginning and endpoint of each interval.

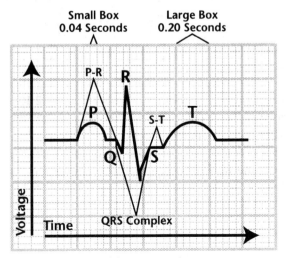

*Fig. 1-6. Components of the ECG waveforms.*

The first interval in the cardiac cycle is the **P-R interval**. The **P-R interval** represents the transmission of an electrical impulse from the SA node through the atria and AV junction. A normal **P-R interval** indicates that conduction from the SA node through the AV junction is free of obstruction or delays. Also, a normal **P-R interval** implies that the atrial chambers have had sufficient time to pump blood into the ventricles.

The second interval that requires evaluation is the **S-T segment**. The **S-T segment** represents the start of the *repolarization* of the ventricles. The **S-T segment** begins with the completion of the QRS complex and ends with the beginning of the T wave. A normal **S-T segment** is flat and relatively close to the baseline (also called the isoelectric line). An **S-T segment** that is significantly above or below the baseline may indicate myocardial ischemia, previous myocardial infarction, cardiac disease or effects of certain medications.

The **R-R interval** represents the time from one cardiac cycle to the next cycle. The **R-R interval** is measured from the peak of any given **R wave** to the peak of the next **R wave**. The heart rate directly effects the **R-R interval**. For example, the faster the heart rate, the shorter the **R-R interval**. Measure and compare at least three **R-R intervals** within the rhythm to determine if the rhythm is regular or irregular. (see Figs. 1-7a, 1-7b)

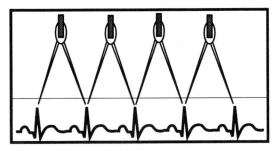

*Fig. 1-7a. Regular R-R intervals.*

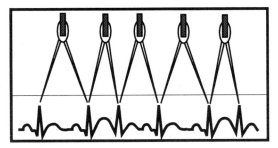

*Figs. 1-7b. Irregular R-R intervals.*

### Etiologies of Dysrhythmias

ECG dysrhythmias may be benign or life threatening. Dysrhythmias may arise from acute and reversible causes such as inadequate oxygenation. Other dysrhythmias are chronic and may be the result of extensive damage to the myocardial tissue and conduction system. Some acute and chronic conditions include:

- coronary artery disease
- myocardial ischemia
- myocardial infarction

- digitalis toxicity
- fear, anxiety, or emotional stress
- electrolyte imbalance
- stimulants, i.e., caffeine, nicotine, etc.
- left- or right-sided heart failure
- hypoxemia or acidosis
- drug overdose
- cardiomyopathies
- post open heart surgery
- rheumatic fever
- electrical shock
- blunt or penetrating chest trauma
- right or left ventricular hypertrophy
- metabolic conditions, i.e., thyroid, anemia
- chronic obstructive pulmonary disease
- valvular disease
- medications including:
  - catecholamines
  - beta blockers
  - calcium channel blockers
  - antiarrhythmics

## Interpretation Tools

ECG paper is marked with a grid to provide a guide for measuring the amplitude and length of the waveforms and intervals. Standard ECG paper is composed of **small boxes** of **.04 seconds** each, and **large boxes** consisting of 5 small boxes that total **.20 seconds** each. The large boxes are inscribed with a heavier line. Five consecutive **large boxes** equal **one second**. Most ECG paper is marked at the top with a vertical slash or an arrow indicating three-second intervals. Each of these time intervals is helpful in determining the heart rate. The ECG recorder is set at a standard speed of **25 mm per second.** The tracing on the ECG graph paper is produced by a heated stylus that literally burns the waveforms onto the paper. The stylus moves up and down on the graph paper in response to the electrical stimulus received.

### ECG Leads

Electrical impulses traveling through the cardiac conduction system can be monitored by attaching electrodes to the surface of the skin. Electrical impulses traveling toward the *positive* electrode will result in an *upward* deflection on the ECG paper. (see Fig. 1-8) An

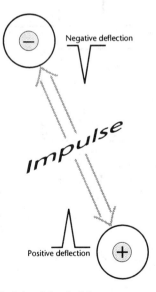

*Fig. 1-8. Principles of electrical flow.*

impulse traveling toward the *negative* electrode will
result in a *downward* deflection on the ECG paper.
When there is no electrical activity in the heart, or if
the electrical forces are equal, the ECG tracing will
show a flat line. This line is called the *isoelectric line,* or
baseline, and is used as a reference point to evaluate the
waveforms. The *ground* electrode is a safety feature that
has a zero electrical potential. The *ground* lead helps to
eliminate extraneous electrical interference from enter-
ing the monitor circuit.

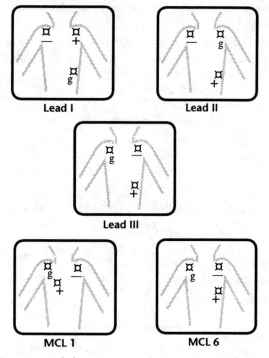

*Fig. 1-9. Lead placement.*

The heart can be viewed from twelve different aspects, or leads. The most commonly used leads for field or routine bedside monitoring are leads I, II, III, MCL1 and MCL6. These leads can be established by arranging a positive, negative and a ground lead in the configurations shown in Fig. 1-9.

Each lead accentuates certain parts of the tracing. It is best to find a lead that will give you a clear tracing with prominent waveforms. Lead II and MCL1 are the most commonly used continuous monitoring leads as they typically provide the most information about the waveforms and intervals. The *EZ ECG* program displays all of the ECG rhythms in lead II.

Occasionally you may have difficulty getting a clear tracing on the ECG paper. Any marking on the ECG paper that is not directly related to cardiac conduction is called **artifact.** Many factors can contribute to **artifact.** Fig. 1-10 lists troubleshooting tips for reducing outside interference. In some cases **artifact** may mimic a life-threatening dysrhythmia. Therefore, it is important to always eliminate the possibility of **artifact** and check your patient's status prior to treating any dysrhythmia.

### Rate Calculation

An important part of interpreting ECG rhythms is to determine the **heart rate.** Heart rate is often a factor used to determine if a patient is stable or unstable. It is also an important criterion for choosing medications or electrical therapy. A heart that is beating **too slow** may not be pumping enough blood to supply the body's needs. When the heart is beating **too fast** the ventricles and coronary arteries do not have sufficient time to adequately fill. This results in a decreased cardiac output.

A concept to always remember is that each QRS complex should generate a **pulse.** The only way to determine if each QRS complex is corresponding to actual movement of blood through the heart is to take a **pulse** and simultaneously watch the ECG monitor.

Most of the newer ECG monitoring machines are equipped with an electronic digital display of the heart rate. This is only helpful during actual "live" monitor-

---

Artifacts are distortions that obscure the cardiac impulse on the ECG tracing. Artifact may be caused by electrical, mechanical or patient interference. This often makes accurate interpretation difficult. Artifact may appear similar to a life-threatening dysrhythmia. Remember, the "patient is always right." Be sure to check the status of your patient before initiating any electrical or drug therapy. Listed below are a few tips for eliminating unwanted artifact:

| *Patient Preparation:* | *Check for and correct:* |
|---|---|
| Explain procedure | Amplitude of gain |
| Preserve modesty | Lead selection |
| Dry skin | Dry electrode gel |
| Remove hair | Loose electrodes |
| Gently abrade and clean skin | Lead wire connection |
| Insure personal and patient safety | Damage to lead wires |
| | Improper electrode placement |
| | Patient movement |
| | T wave amplitude greater than R wave |
| | 60-cycle interference |

*Fig. 1-10. ECG troubleshooting.*

ing of a patient with a corresponding pulse. You may not always be able to rely on the monitor and will have to determine the heart rate using the ECG strip. There are many methods and shortcuts for determining the heart rate using the ECG graph paper and frequency of the cardiac cycles.

The quickest, and most simple method is to count the number of R waves found in a six second strip and multiply by 10, as seen in Fig. 1-11. This will provide you with a "ballpark" estimate of the rate per minute.

Keep in mind that in some dysrhythmias, the rates of the atria and ventricles may differ. In other words, the P waves may have a different rate than the QRS complexes. When this occurs, you will need to calculate the rate of each.

There are two calculation methods that involve evaluating the R-R interval. The first is the **triplicate method,** which is only considered accurate if the over-

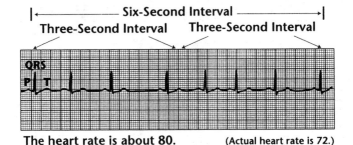

**The heart rate is about 80.**          (Actual heart rate is 72.)

*Fig. 1-11. Three- and six-second intervals. (From Huszar RJ: Basic dysrhythmias: interpretation and management, 2e, St. Louis, 1994, Mosby.)*

all rhythm is regular. To use this method:

1.  Select an R wave that lands on a dark vertical line on the ECG paper.

2.  Count the "big boxes" from left to right. Memorize the numbers 300, 150, 100, 75, 60, and 50 consecutively.

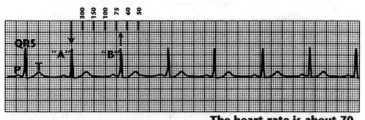

The heart rate is about 70.

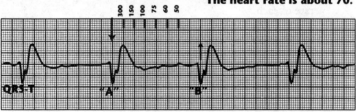

The heart rate is less than 50.

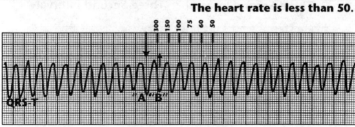

The heart rate is about 250.

*Fig. 1-12. Triplicate method. (From Huszar RJ. Basic dysrhythmias, interpretation and management, 2e, St. Louis, 1994, Mosby.)*

3. You may need to estimate the rate if the second R wave lands in the middle of a "big box." (See the examples in Fig. 1-12.)

Another method that uses the R-R interval to determine heart rate requires you to use a **conversion table.** Count the number of small (0.04 sec) boxes between R waves and refer to the rate conversion table below, Fig. 1-13. This will provide you with an accurate heart rate. The only drawback to this method is that the **conversion table** must be memorized or available for reference each time you need to determine the heart rate.

## *Five Step Rhythm Analysis*

| Small Boxes | Heart Rate Per Minute | Small Boxes | Heart Rate Per Minute |
|---|---|---|---|
| 4 | – 375 | 21 | – 71 |
| 5 | – 300 | 22 | – 68 |
| 6 | – 250 | 23 | – 65 |
| 7 | – 214 | 24 | – 63 |
| 8 | – 188 | 25 | – 60 |
| 9 | – 167 | 26 | – 58 |
| 10 | – 150 | 28 | – 54 |
| 11 | – 136 | 30 | – 50 |
| 12 | – 125 | 32 | – 47 |
| 13 | – 115 | 34 | – 44 |
| 14 | – 107 | 36 | – 42 |
| 15 | – 100 | 38 | – 40 |
| 16 | – 94 | 40 | – 38 |
| 17 | – 88 | 42 | – 36 |
| 18 | – 83 | 44 | – 34 |
| 19 | – 79 | 48 | – 31 |
| 20 | – 75 | 50 | – 30 |

*Fig. 1-13. Rate conversion table.*

At first glance some ECG rhythms may be intimidating. By approaching each rhythm strip using the **five step rhythm analysis method** you will soon become proficient at evaluating the criteria necessary to identify most rhythms. The five steps are:

1. Calculate the **QRS rate**
2. Assess the **regularity** of the rhythm
3. Evaluate the **atrial activity**
4. Determine the **QRS width**
5. Observe the **P to QRS relationship**

1. Calculate the **rate** of the QRS complexes. If you are bedside with the patient it is important to check the pulse and determine if it correlates with the QRS rate. If there are more or less P waves than QRS complexes then also calculate the rate of the P waves.

2. Observe the **rhythm** for at least 20 to 30 seconds and determine if the rhythm is regular or irregular. Most authorities agree that the R-R intervals may vary as much as 0.04 seconds for the rhythm to still be considered regular.

3. The P wave reflects the **atrial activity**. Compare the appearance and configuration of the P waves.

4. Measure the **width of the QRS complex**. A normal QRS complex is less than 0.12 seconds (or three little boxes) wide. A QRS complex wider than 0.12 seconds may be the result of a block located in the bundle branches. (Some authorities state the QRS complex should be ≤0.10 sec-

onds.) A wide QRS complex may also indicate
that the source of the rhythm is a ventricular
impulse.

5. Observe the **relationship between the P waves
and the QRS complexes.** Normally, there
should only be one P wave for each QRS complex. Some dysrhythmias may have more P
waves than QRS complexes. Next, measure the
P-R interval. A normal P-R interval will be
between 0.12 and 0.20 seconds (or three to five
little boxes) long.

## Important Terminology

Interpretation of ECGs includes communicating your findings with other healthcare personnel and documenting your interpretations. Knowledge of the terminology to most accurately describe ECG rhythms will facilitate these communications. Read through all of the words in this guide and learn the terms that are new to you. You can also use this section as a glossary/dictionary. This list is only a partial compilation of ECG terms, so you may need to refer to an ECG text or medical dictionary for words not included in this list.

**Antiarrhythmic** - refers to medications that attempt to prevent or decrease the frequency of dysrhythmias and ectopic impulses.

**Arteriosclerosis** - hardening and loss of elasticity of the arteries.

**Asystole** - absence of electrical activity and contraction of the heart.

**Atherosclerosis** - a condition caused by an accumulation of debris along the intimal layer of the arteries.

**Atrial kick** - filling of the ventricles with blood as a result of complete contraction of the atria.

**AV block** - partial or complete obstruction of electrical impulses through the atrioventricular node. AV blocks are categorized as first-, second-, or third-degree.

**Bigeminy** - ectopic complexes occurring every other complex.

**Bradycardia** - a slow heart rate, less than 60 beats per minute.

**Cardiac cycle** - includes the systolic and diastolic phases of the heart beat. A normal cycle includes the P, Q, R, S, and T waveforms.

**Cardiac output** - the amount of blood pumped by the heart in one minute.

**Compensatory pause** - a pause following a premature complex which allows the SA node to continue at its preset rhythm.

**Conductivity** - the property of cardiac cells to transmit electrical impulses.

**Contractility** - the ability of the cardiac cells to shorten when stimulated.

**Controlled** - the ventricular rate is considered controlled if it is less than 100 beats per minute.

**Couplet** - two consecutive PVCs.

**Depolarization** - the electrical process of discharging a resting cardiac cell.

**Diastole** - the period of relaxation of the atria and ventricles. It is during this phase when the chambers of the heart and coronary arteries fill with blood.

**Dysrhythmia** - any ECG rhythm other than the normal sinus rhythm. May be benign or lethal.

**Ectopic** - a beat or rhythm originating from a site other than the SA node. Ectopic beats are often premature.

**Escape** - a complex or rhythm that is initiated when the underlying rhythm slows to less than the escape pacemaker's inherent rate.

**Fibrillation** - chaotic, uncoordinated electrical activity within the myocardium producing a quivering, ineffective muscular activity.

**Flutter** - a regular pattern of electrical activity which displays a saw-tooth appearance on the ECG.

**Ground** - electrode with a zero electrical potential that helps eliminate extraneous electrical interference.

**Hemodynamic** - forces involved in perfusing the body with blood. Includes factors such as heart rate, force, preload, afterload and vessel tone.

**Hypertrophy** - enlargement of a portion of the heart without an increase in chamber size.

**Idioventricular** - rhythm originating within the ventricles.

**Infarction** - necrotic tissue due to a sustained period of interrupted blood flow.

**Inherent** - the rate at which a dominant or escape pacemaker normally initiates impulses.

**Interval** - measurable segments between ECG waveforms.

**Ischemia** - reduction in flow of oxygenated blood to a portion of cardiac tissue which may be transient or irreversible.

**Isoelectric** - a flat line on the ECG indicating no electrical activity or variations.

**Joule** - a unit of electrical energy delivered through the chest wall for the purpose of synchronized cardioversion or defibrillation of the heart.

**Junctional** - a term used to describe ectopic or escape rhythms originating within the AV junction.

**Mobitz** - name of the physician who identified two types of second-degree AV block.

**Multifocal** - term used to describe impulses that originate from multiple ectopic locations.

**Myocardium** - pertaining to the heart muscle.

**Necrosis** - dead tissue from an insufficient supply of oxygenated blood.

**Parasympathetic** - the portion of the autonomic nervous system that produces slowing and depressing of cardiac function.

**Paroxysmal** - abrupt onset of a dysrhythmia.

**Perfusion** - flow of blood to tissues and/or organs.

**Pulseless Electrical Activity** - electrical activity displayed on the ECG without evidence of mechanical response (no pulse).

**Purkinje fibers** - the terminal portion of the cardiac conduction system imbedded within the ventricles.

**Quadrigeminy** - ectopic beat occurring every fourth complex.

**Reentry** - a circuit of ectopic beats caused by a single electrical impulse returning to a portion of tissue for a second or subsequent time.

**Refractory** - inability to respond to an electrical stimulus due to incomplete repolarization.

**Repolarization** - the process by which a cell is restored to an electrically ready state.

**Sinus** - pertaining to rhythms generated by the dominant pacemaker of the heart—the sinus node.

**Supraventricular** - refers to the portion of the heart from above the bundle branches to the SA node.

**Sympathetic** - the division of the autonomic nervous system responsible for stimulating cardiac activity.

**Synchronize** - an electrical shock timed to depolarize the entire myocardium. The shock is timed to coincide with the R wave to prevent depolarization during the vulnerable T wave.

**Systole** - contraction and subsequent movement of blood through the heart.

**Tachycardia** - a rapid heart rate, typically greater than 100 beats per minute.

**Trigeminy** - an ectopic complex arising every third beat.

**Uncontrolled** - a term used to describe a rhythm with a ventricular response greater than 100 beats per minute.

**Unifocal** - arising from a single ectopic focus.

**Vagal** - refers to the tenth cranial (vagus) nerve that influences heart rate and AV node conduction time by regulating parasympathetic tone.

**Voltage** - the height and depth of a waveform measured in millimeters.

**Watt/second** - see joules.

**Wenckebach** - the name of the physician credited with discovering second-degree AV block type I.

## *Standard ECG Abbreviations*

**AIVR** - accelerated idioventricular rhythm

**AV** - atrioventricular

**BBB** - bundle branch block

**DC** - direct current

**ECG** - electrocardiogram

**EKG** - electrocardiogram (German abbrev.)

**EMD** - electromechanical dissociation (see PEA)

**f wave** - fibrillatory wave

**F wave** - flutter wave

**IVR** - idioventricular rhythm

**LBBB** - left bundle branch block

**MCL** - modified chest lead

**mV** - millivolt

**NSR** - normal sinus rhythm (see RSR)

**PAC** - premature atrial complex

**PAT** - paroxysmal atrial tachycardia

**PEA** - pulseless electrical activity

**PJC** - premature junctional complex

**PJT** - paroxysmal junctional tachycardia

**PVC** - premature ventricular complex

**RSR** - regular sinus rhythm

**RBBB** - right bundle branch block

**SA** - sinoatrial

**SVT** - supraventricular tachycardia

**VF** - ventricular fibrillation

**VT** - ventricular tachycardia

**WAP** - wandering atrial pacemaker

**1°AVBL** - first-degree AV block

**2°AVBL** - second-degree AV block type I or type II

**3°AVBL** - third-degree AV block

# SECTION 2

## SINUS RHYTHMS
### *Normal Sinus Rhythm*
### *Sinus Bradycardia*
### *Sinus Arrhythmia*
### *Sinus Tachycardia*
### *Sinus Pause*

## SINUS RHYTHMS

Standards have been established that define specific parameters for determining normal cardiac conduction. These standards include rates, waveform configurations, and intervals that are considered within "normal" limits for a healthy heart. The **normal sinus rhythm** is the basis, or reference point by which all other rhythms are compared.

All of the sinus rhythms originate from the dominant pacemaker, the **sinus node.** Rhythms originating from outside the sinus node can be placed into one of three categories. The categories are defined by their location of origin and are labeled **atrial, junctional,** or **ventricular.**

Any rhythm that does not meet the criteria for normal sinus rhythm is called a **dysrhythmia.** The term dysrhythmia implies that there is a disturbance within the cardiac conduction system. Dysrhythmias have many implications including; acute or chronic cardiac disease, or myocardial damage. The term **arrhythmia** is often used synonymously with the term dysrhythmia, although the term arrhythmia literally means the absence of any rhythm. Section Three covers each dysrhythmia in detail.

This section will define the criteria for rhythms originating from the sinus node. Rhythm strip examples of the following rhythms will be shown in lead II:

- Normal Sinus Rhythm
- Sinus Bradycardia
- Sinus Arrhythmia
- Sinus Tachycardia
- Sinus Pause

Throughout the booklet, each rhythm will be broken down into the categories used in the **five step rhythm analysis method.** It is important to use this systematic approach with each rhythm you analyze. By using a standard and consistent method with every ECG rhythm you encounter, you will avoid missing any of the critical elements of the rhythm.

NORMAL SINUS RHYTHM

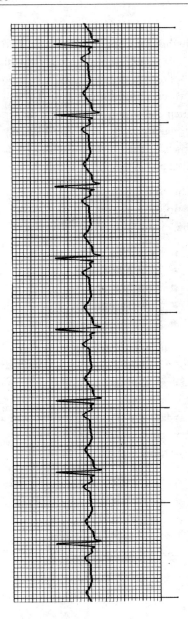

## CRITERIA

*Normal Sinus Rhythm,* sometimes also called regular sinus rhythm, indicates that the pacing impulse is initiated within the sinus node and is transmitted normally down the conduction pathway.

*QRS Rate* 60 to 100 beats per minute.

*Rhythm* Regular.

*Atrial Activity* Normal and consistent P wave configuration.

*QRS Width* 0.04 to 0.12 seconds.

*P to QRS Relationship* 1:1 relationship with a P-R interval between 0.12 and 0.20 seconds.

*Treatment* When associated with a pulse, generally no treatment required.

---

The "**3 to 5 Rule**" states that a
**Normal Sinus Rhythm**
will have between:

3 to 5 small boxes in each P-R interval

3 to 5 large boxes in each R-R interval

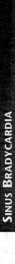

SINUS BRADYCARDIA

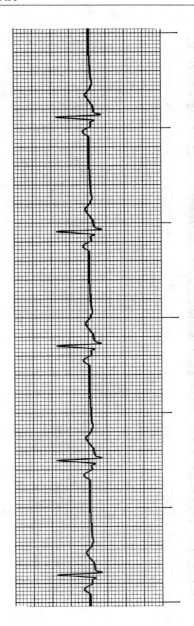

## CRITERIA

*Sinus Bradycardia* may be a normal rhythm in individuals with healthy hearts. *Sinus bradycardia* may also be a sign of acute or chronic heart disease, or it may be caused by an adverse reaction to medications that decrease the heart rate.

*QRS Rate* Less than 60 beats per minute.

*Rhythm* Regular.

*Atrial Activity* Normal and consistent P wave configuration.

*QRS Width* 0.04 to 0.12 seconds.

*P to QRS Relationship* 1:1 relationship with a P-R interval between 0.12 and 0.20 seconds.

*Treatment* Treatment is based on symptoms. If the patient is symptomatic of inadequate cardiac output, medications to increase heart rate such as atropine may be administered. In some situations a pacemaker may be required.

SINUS ARRHYTHMIA

## CRITERIA

*Sinus Arrhythmia* is a variation of normal sinus rhythm. It is common in children, healthy young adults, and the elderly. *Sinus arrhythmia* is usually caused by an inhibition of the vagus (parasympathetic) nerve during inspiration. A rhythmic pattern can be observed of an increase in heart rate during inspiration and a decrease in rate during expiration.

*QRS Rate* Usually 60 to 100 per minute.

*Rhythm* Irregular.

*Atrial Activity* Normal and consistent P wave configuration.

*QRS Width* 0.04 to 0.12 seconds.

*P to QRS Relationship* 1:1 relationship with a P-R interval between 0.12 and 0.20 seconds.

*Treatment* Usually no treatment is required unless the rate is slow and producing symptoms of inadequate cardiac output. In such cases atropine may be given to increase conduction through the AV node, or a pacemaker may be applied.

**SINUS TACHYCARDIA**

## CRITERIA

*Sinus Tachycardia* is typically caused by an increase in the body's need for oxygenated blood such as during physical exertion, dehydration, fever, or shock. *Sinus tachycardia* may be a response to pain or fear. Occasionally, *sinus tachycardia* may be due to a myocardial infarction or congestive heart failure.

*QRS Rate* 100 to 150 beats per minute.

*Rhythm* Regular.

*Atrial Activity* Normal and consistent P wave configuration.

*QRS Width* 0.04 to 0.12 seconds.

*P to QRS Relationship* 1:1 relationship with a P-R interval between 0.12 and 0.20 seconds.

*Treatment* Treatment should be focused on correcting the underlying cause. Oxygen therapy may be beneficial.

SINUS PAUSE

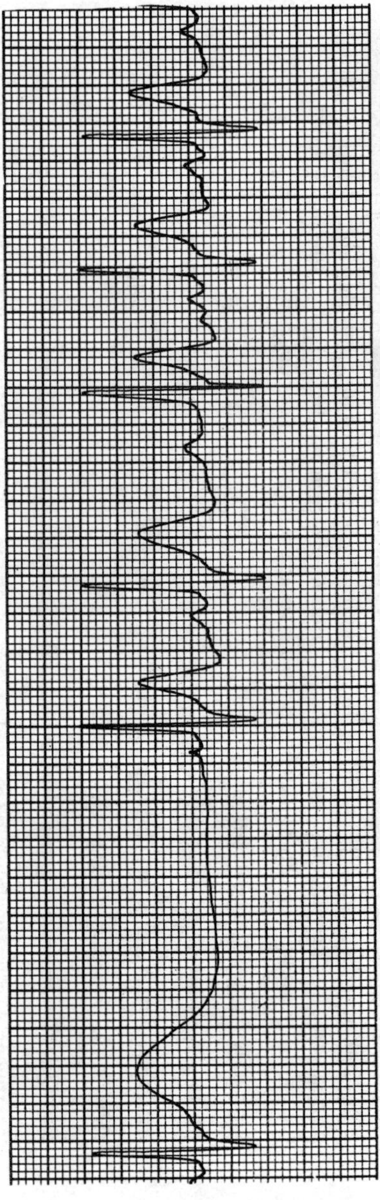

## CRITERIA

*Sinus Pause* may occur as a result of transient ischemia or permanent damage to the SA node. *Sinus pause* may also be caused by increase vagal (parasympathetic) tone, electrolyte imbalance or an adverse effect of certain medications. The sinus node may fail to fire for one or more complexes.

*QRS Rate* Usually 60 to 100, but may vary.

*Rhythm* Irregular due to the pause (the underlying rhythm is often regular).

*Atrial Activity* Normal and consistent P wave configuration in the underlying rhythm. (Note: The rhythm after a pause may be an escape beat or rhythm.)

*QRS Width* 0.04 to 0.12 seconds.

*P to QRS Relationship* 1:1 relationship with a P-R interval of 0.12 to 0.20 seconds when sinus beats are present.

*Treatment* Usually no treatment is indicated unless the patient shows signs of low cardiac output. Further observation is advised.

## DYSRHYTHMIAS

*Ectopic Beats and Rhythms*
*Atrioventricular Blocks*
*Escape Rhythms*

## DYSRHYTHMIAS

Now that you have an understanding of the rhythms that originate from the sinus node, let's move on to rhythms that are abnormally conducted. Disturbances in cardiac conduction are called **dysrhythmias**. Dysrhythmias can occur even in healthy hearts. Often minor dysrhythmias produce no symptoms and resolve without any treatment. More serious dysrhythmias indicate significant acute or chronic heart disease. When serious dysrhythmias occur medication is often required to either speed up or slow down the ventricular rate, or to suppress an irritable area within the myocardium. Occasionally, surgical intervention or thrombolytic therapy is needed to prevent further damage and salvage any remaining viable heart tissue. Dysrhythmias that are too fast or completely chaotic may respond to the electrical therapy of synchronized cardioversion or defibrillation.

Once a dysrhythmia has been identified, it is important to carefully assess the patient's vital signs and general cardiovascular status. You must determine how well the patient is tolerating the rhythm and how aggressively the dysrhythmia should be treated.

Dysrhythmias can be evaluated from three viewpoints.

1. The first way is to evaluate the ventricular response. The contraction of the ventricles determines the majority of the cardiac output and perfusion of blood to the tissues. The ventricular response can be assessed by palpating for a pulse during the QRS complexes. Abnormal conduction can viewed as being:

- Too fast
- Too slow
- Too irritable
- Lethal or absent

2. Dysrhythmias are placed into categories based on the origin of the impulse formation. The prefix of the dysrhythmia will identify the origin as either:

- Atrial
- Junctional
- Ventricular

3. Another way dysrhythmias are categorized is by the electrophysiology of the conduction disturbance. The *EZ ECGs* booklet places the dysrhythmias into groups based on similar distinguishing traits. The dysrhythmias will be categorized as:

- Ectopic beats
- Ectopic rhythms
- Atrioventricular blocks
- Escape rhythms

The five step rhythm analysis method will be applied to each dysrhythmia example.

### Ectopic Beats and Rhythms

An abnormal impulse formation may initiate an **ectopic beat or rhythm**. The three predominant mechanisms that generate ectopic beats and rhythms are:

- Reentry
- Enhanced Automaticity
- Triggered Activity

*Reentry* occurs when an electrical impulse is blocked or delayed in a portion of the conduction system. The interruption of impulses allow some of the unaffected cells time to repolarize. Once repolarized, the cells can be depolarized a subsequent time. (see Fig. 3-1) This may result in a single (ectopic) beat or repetitive abnormal impulses (ectopic rhythm) which are often tachycardic. Reentry is commonly caused by ischemic heart disease, myocardial infarction, or electrolyte imbalances.

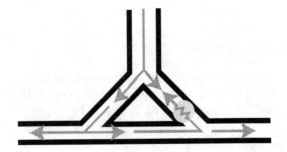

*Fig. 3-1. Reentry.*

*Enhanced automaticity* occurs when impulses from the pacemaker cells are altered. This causes either an enhancement of impulses from normal pacemaker cells, or conflicting impulses arising from the same pacemaker site. The alteration and interference of impulses causes ectopic beats and rhythms. Enhanced automaticity may be caused by hypoxia, digitalis toxicity, electrolyte imbalances, ischemic heart disease, myocardial infarction, cardio-myopathies, or actions of cardiac medications.

*Triggered activity* occurs when pacemaker and/or non-pacemaker cells depolarize multiple times following a single electrical stimulation. Triggered activity is the result of "after depolarizations" that occur immediately after a cardiac cycle, or just before the next cycle. This type of abnormal conduction can result in ectopic beats, runs of beats or paroxysmal tachycardias. The causes of triggered activity are similar to those causing enhanced automaticity.

Understanding the electrophysiology behind a dysrhythmia is not as important as being able to correctly identify the rhythm and knowing the appropriate interventions for each. Remember, most of the life-threatening, lethal dysrhythmias are the easiest to identify.

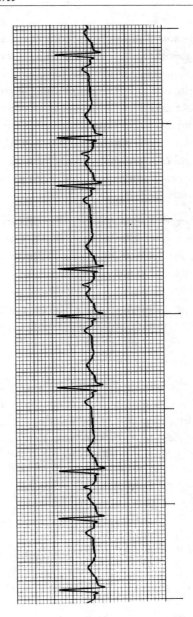

## CRITERIA

*Premature Atrial Complexes*, abbreviated PACs, are isolated early beats that indicate an irritable focus within the atria. *Premature atrial complexes* may appear in healthy hearts or may indicate disease or damage within the atrial tissue. Often PACs are caused by stimulants such as emotional stress, caffeine, or nicotine.

*QRS Rate* May occur at any heart rate.

*Rhythm* Irregular when PACs occur.

*Atrial Activity* P waves may or may not be seen preceding the ectopic complex.

*QRS Width* The QRS width is not usually affected by a PAC and will appear similar to the QRS complexes in the underlying rhythm.

*P to QRS Relationship* 1:1 relationship for all complexes with observable P waves.

*Treatment* Often no treatment is required. Remove suspect stimulants. Evaluate for underlying heart disease and treat accordingly.

PREMATURE JUNCTIONAL COMPLEXES

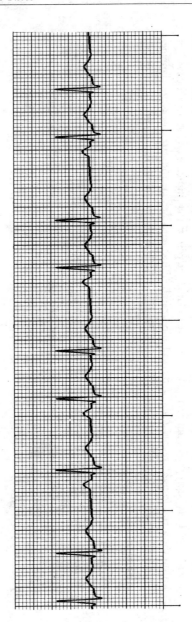

## CRITERIA

*Premature Junctional Complexes,* abbreviated PJCs, are isolated early beats that indicate an irritable focus within the AV junction. PJCs may occur in healthy individuals without any obvious cause, but may be caused by disease involving the tissues of the AV junction. Certain medications may cause PJCs, most commonly digitalis.

*QRS Rate* May occur at any heart rate.

*Rhythm* Irregular when PJCs occur.

*Atrial Activity* P waves may appear before or after the QRS of the ectopic complex, or may be hidden within the QRS.

*QRS Width* The QRS width is not usually affected by a PJC and will appear similar to the QRS complexes in the underlying rhythm.

*P to QRS Relationship* 1:1 relationship for all complexes with observable P waves.

*Treatment* Often no treatment is required. Check for digitalis toxicity or other medications in non-therapeutic doses.

PREMATURE VENTRICULAR COMPLEXES

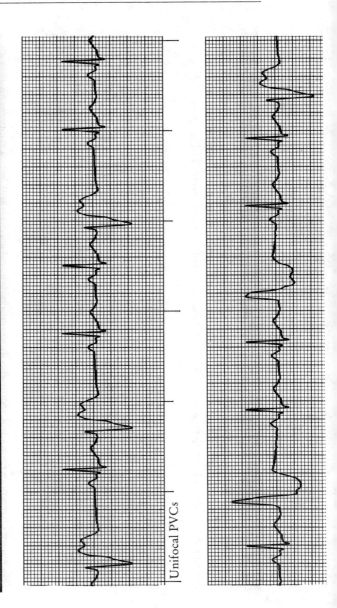

Unifocal PVCs

| Multifocal PVCs |

## CRITERIA

*Premature Ventricular Complexes,* also called PVCs, are early beats that indicate one or more irritable foci within the ventricles. PVCs that are similar in appearance indicate a single area of irritability and are called **unifocal** PVCs. PVCs that are different in appearance indicate more than one area of irritability and are called **multifocal** PVCs. PVCs may occur in healthy individuals and should not cause concern. PVCs often indicate ischemic heart disease, hypoxia, electrolyte imbalances, myocardial infarction, or an adverse response to certain medications.

*QRS Rate* PVCs may occur at any heart rate.

*Rhythm* Irregular when PVCs occur.

*Atrial Activity* P waves may or may not be seen preceding the ectopic complex.

*QRS Width* The hallmark of PVCs is a QRS complex that is greater than 0.12 seconds.

*P to QRS Relationship* There is no observable relationship between the P waves and the QRS complexes of PVCs.

*Treatment* Treatment of PVCs is based on the frequency and focus of the PVCs, as well as the presence of any associated symptoms. Treatment often includes antiarrhythmic drugs such as lidocaine and oxygen administration.

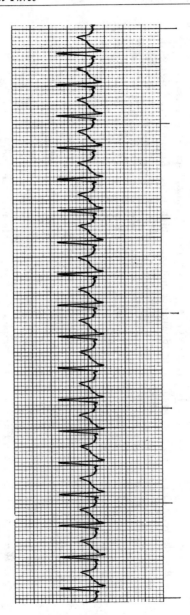

ATRIAL TACHYCARDIA

## CRITERIA

*Atrial Tachycardia* originates from an irritable focus within the atria. *Atrial tachycardia* frequently has an abrupt onset. This is called paroxysmal atrial tachycardia (PAT). *Atrial tachycardia* is considered a supraventricular tachycardia (SVT or PSVT when paroxysmal). *Atrial tachycardia* is usually caused by ischemic heart disease, a myocardial infarction, or digitalis toxicity. Patients with *atrial tachycardia* often complain of feelings of palpitations or a fluttering sensation in their chest.

*QRS Rate* 160 to 250.

*Rhythm* Regular.

*Atrial Activity* P waves may or may not be visible.

*QRS Width* 0.04 to 0.12 seconds.

*P to QRS Relationship* Any visible P waves will have usually have a 1:1 relationship with the QRS complexes.

*Treatment* Treatment may include vagal maneuvers, medications such as adenosine or verapamil and/or synchronized cardioversion.

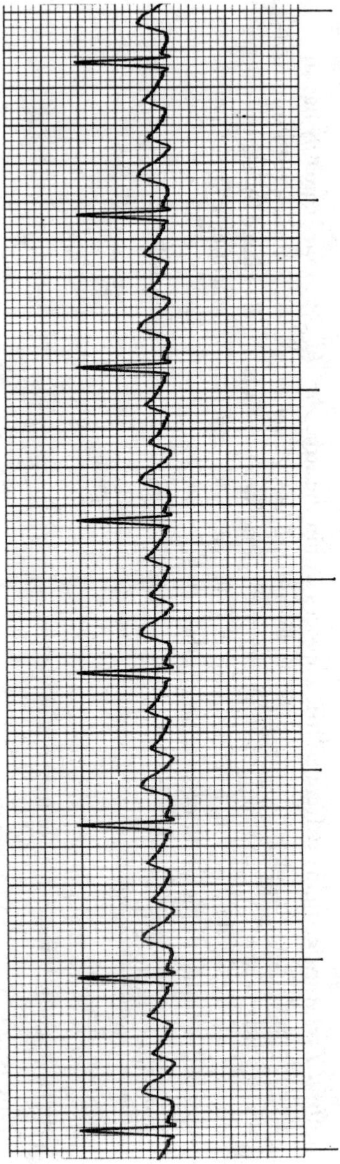

## CRITERIA

*Atrial Flutter* is most often caused by a reentry circuit within the atria. The identifying feature of this rhythm is the "picket-fence" or "saw-tooth" pattern F waves between the QRS complexes. The fluttering within the atria does not allow for complete emptying of the atrial chambers into the ventricles. This results in a reduction of about 25% of the cardiac output. *Atrial flutter* is seen in patients with rheumatic heart disease, valvular problems and ischemic disease.

*QRS Rate* May vary from slow to tachycardic. A rate below 100 per minute is labeled "controlled," above 100 per minute is "uncontrolled."

*Rhythm* The atrial F waves will be regular. QRS rhythm may be regular or irregular.

*Atrial Activity* Characteristic F waves with a rate of 250 to 350 per minute.

*QRS Width* Usually normal at 0.04 to 0.12 seconds. F waves may coincide with some of the QRS complexes causing some complexes to appear distorted.

*P to QRS Relationship* F waves replace normal P waves and may have a 2:1, 3:1, or 4:1 relationship.

*Treatment* Treatment is based on the QRS rate and may include digitalis or cardioversion.

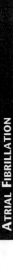

ATRIAL FIBRILLATION

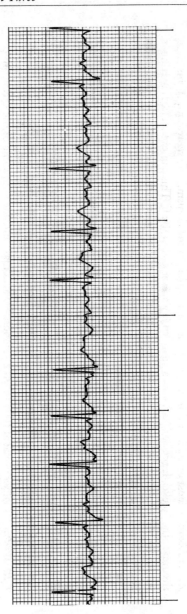

## CRITERIA

*Atrial Fibrillation* is caused by enhanced automaticity or a reentry mechanism. The chaotic unorganized electrical activity within the atria cause the chambers to quiver ineffectively. This can reduce the cardiac output by as much as 25%. *Atrial fibrillation* is common in the elderly and individuals with coronary artery disease. It is frequently associated with congestive heart failure.

*QRS Rate* The QRS rate may be "controlled" at less than 100 per minute, or "uncontrolled" at greater than 100 beats per minute.

*Rhythm* The QRS rhythm is typically irregular.

*Atrial Activity* No discernible P waves. Atrial activity shows chaotic wavy "f waves."

*QRS Width* 0.04 to 0.12 seconds.

*P to QRS Relationship* None.

*Treatment* Treatment is based on the rate of the ventricular response and may include drugs such as digitalis, beta blockers, or synchronized cardioversion.

VENTRICULAR TACHYCARDIA

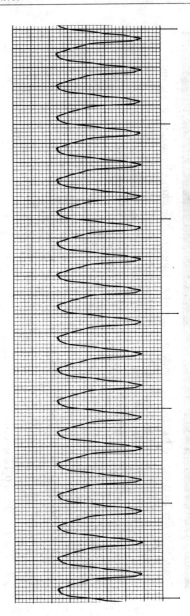

## CRITERIA

*Ventricular Tachycardia (V-tach)* is caused by an irritable focus within the Purkinje fibers or ventricular myocardium. Three or more PVCs in a row is considered *ventricular tachycardia*. *V-tach* may be attributed to hypoxia, electrolyte imbalances, or significant heart disease. *V-tach* is an ominous, life threatening dysrhythmia that requires rapid intervention. Without treatment *V-tach* may quickly decline into V-fib.

*QRS Rate* 100 to 250 per minute.

*Rhythm* Usually regular.

*Atrial Activity* P waves may or may not be present.

*QRS Width* Greater than 0.12 seconds.

*P to QRS Relationship* None.

*Treatment* Treatment for V-tach is based on whether or not a pulse is present. If a pulse is present treatment is based upon the patient's hemodynamic status. Antiarrhythmic medications such as lidocaine, procainamide or bretylium may be administered. Other treatments may include synchronized cardioversion, defibrillation and CPR.

VENTRICULAR FIBRILLATION

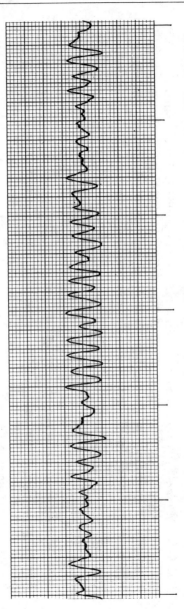

## CRITERIA

*Ventricular Fibrillation (V-fib)* occurs when the cells of the ventricular myocardium depolarize in a chaotic and uncoordinated manner. No pulse can be felt during *ventricular fibrillation* as the heart is incapable of pumping blood. Causes of *V-fib* include acute myocardial infarction, electrolyte imbalances, hypoxia and adverse reactions to medications.

*QRS Rate* None.

*Rhythm* Chaotic.

*Atrial Activity* None.

*QRS Width* No discernable complexes can be observed. Fibrillatory waves may be coarse (large) or fine (small).

*P to QRS Relationship* None.

*Treatment* Rapid defibrillation is the treatment of choice. CPR should be initiated until a defibrillator is available. Medications may include epinephrine, antiarrhythmics and magnesium sulfate. Note: loose leads, patient movement or artifact may mimic V-fib, therefore it is important to always check the patient's status, lead attachment, and the monitor prior to implementing treatment.

### *Atrioventricular Blocks*

**Atrioventricular blocks** occur when a portion of the cardiac conduction system is damaged. Ischemic or necrotic tissue can cause delayed or blocked conduction of electrical impulses. AV blocks typically produce slow ventricular rates and treatment is often focused on increasing the heart rate. The key to identifying AV blocks is the P to QRS relationship. By determining the rate of the P waves, the ratio of P waves to QRS complexes and the P-R interval, you will be able to identify the block. AV blocks are placed into three categories based on the location and severity of the block: (see Fig. 3-2)

**First-degree** block is actually not a block but a delay in conduction through the AV node.

**Second-degree** blocks type I and II are more serious AV blocks that are located further down the cardiac conduction system. Second-degree blocks result in missed QRS complexes. This will be seen as dropped QRS complexes or greater than 1:1 ratio of P waves to QRS complexes.

**Third-degree** block, sometimes called complete heart block, indicates that the electrical impulses are completely blocked between the atria and the ventricles. Third-degree block indicates that the ventricles are responding to impulses generated within the lower portion of the AV junction or from the Purkinje fibers in the ventricles.

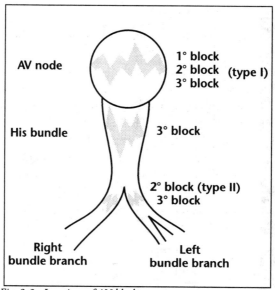

*Fig. 3-2. Locations of AV blocks.*

Another easy way to learn the three classifications of
AV blocks is to remember that in:

**First-Degree AV Block**
"*All* of the beats go through"

**Second-Degree AV Blocks**
"Only *some* of the beats go through"

and

**Third-Degree AV Block**
"*None* of the beats go through"

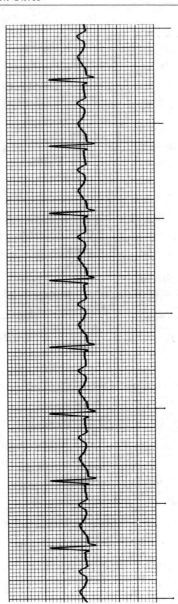

## CRITERIA

*First-Degree AV block* is caused by a delay in conduction through the AV node. *First-degree AV block* may appear in healthy individuals without reason for concern. Other causes of first-degree block include digitalis toxicity, electrolyte imbalances, myocardial ischemia or infarction. Certain medications may cause first-degree AV block by slowing conduction through the AV node.

*QRS Rate* 60 to 100 per minute, occasionally bradycardic and less than 60 per minute.

*Rhythm* Regular.

*Atrial Activity* Normal and consistent P wave configuration.

*QRS Width* 0.04 to 0.12 seconds.

*P to QRS Relationship* 1:1 relationship with a P-R interval greater than .20 seconds.

*Treatment* Usually no treatment is required unless the ventricular rate is less than 60 per minute resulting in an inadequate cardiac output.

SECOND-DEGREE AV BLOCK TYPE I (WENCKEBACH/MOBITZ TYPE I)

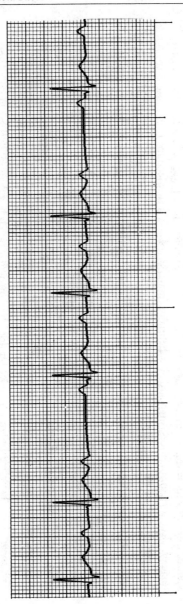

## CRITERIA

*Second-Degree AV Block Type I,* also called Wenckebach or Mobitz Type I, is caused by injury or damage within or just below the AV node. Second-degree type I is most commonly due to an inferior-wall myocardial infarction. Other causes include digitalis toxicity, electrolyte imbalances, ischemic heart disease or post open heart surgery.

*QRS Rate* May occur at any rate.

*Rhythm* Irregular. Note: the hallmark of this rhythm is groups of beats ending with a dropped beat.

*Atrial Activity* Normal and consistent P wave configuration.

*QRS Width* The QRS width is not affected by the block and will be 0.04 to 0.12 seconds.

*P to QRS Relationship* Beginning with each group of beats the P-R interval will progressively lengthen until a QRS complex is dropped. This can be observed by a P wave without a subsequent QRS complex at the end of each group of beats.

*Treatment* Usually no treatment is needed. Treat any underlying cause. If the block is related to an MI it will often resolve within 72 to 96 hours.

SECOND-DEGREE AV BLOCK TYPE II (MOBITZ TYPE II)

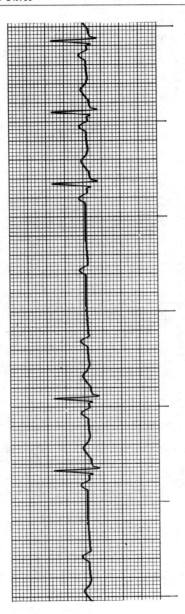

## CRITERIA

*Second-Degree Block Block Type II,* also called Mobitz Type II, is the more serious of the second-degree blocks. This block indicates damage within or below the AV junction with intermittent conduction through the bundle branches. *Second-degree type II* is usually the result of advanced heart disease, although it may be caused by digitalis toxicity. *Second-degree type II* rarely resolves without treatment.

*QRS Rate* May occur at any rate. Most commonly produces slow ventricular rates.

*Rhythm* May be regular or irregular.

*Atrial Activity* Normal and consistent appearing P waves.

*QRS Width* May be normal at 0.04 to 0.12 seconds. If the block is located within the bundle branches the QRS complex may be greater than 0.12 seconds.

*P to QRS Relationship* P waves can be seen that do not conduct QRS complexes. This may occur at regular intervals. i.e., 2:1, 3:1, 4:1 etc. P-R intervals will be constant with all conducted QRS complexes.

*Treatment* Treatment is based on the ventricular rate and cardiac output. This rhythm may not respond well to drugs, and often requires a pacemaker.

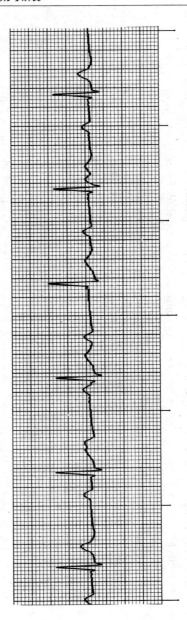

THIRD-DEGREE AV BLOCK (COMPLETE HEART BLOCK)

## CRITERIA

***Third-Degree AV Block,*** also called Complete Heart Block, is the result of a complete blockage of electrical impulses through the AV node and junction. In order for the heart to continue pumping, electrical impulses must be initiated by a junctional or ventricular escape pacemaker. *Third-degree block* with a ventricular escape rhythm is a potentially lethal rhythm which requires immediate action.

***QRS Rate*** The QRS rate is usually less than 60 per minute.

***Rhythm*** Since the atria and ventricles are firing independently, the P waves and QRS complexes will have different rates (the P waves typically will have the faster rate).

***Atrial Activity*** Normal and consistent P wave configuration.

***QRS Width*** The QRS width will depend upon the escape pacemaker and may be normal or wide (>0.12 seconds).

***P to QRS Relationship*** There is no relationship between the P waves and QRS complexes.

***Treatment*** Treatment is based upon the ventricular response rate and cardiac output. This block may not respond to medication and often requires a pacemaker. Close observation is advised.

## Escape Rhythms

Escape rhythms occur when the normal pacemaker, the sinus node, fails to fire or when an impulse is blocked. Escape rhythms may also occur when the AV junction fails to fire at a rate faster than the inherent rate of the ventricles. An escape beat or rhythm may arise after a sinus pause. Third-degree (complete) AV blocks always have either a junctional or ventricular escape rhythm.

The location of the escape rhythm is determined by the ventricular rate and the width of the QRS complexes. Obviously, the slower the rate the greater the potential for decreased cardiac output. Also, the "atrial kick" is lost in escape rhythms further reducing the cardiac output.

Here are some rules to help you to differentiate the escape rhythms:

### Junctional Escape
QRS rate - 40 to 60 per minute
QRS width - narrow

### Ventricular Escape
QRS rate - less than 40 per minute
QRS width - wide

In **junctional escape** rhythms, the P waves may appear before, after or hidden within the QRS complexes. The location of the block and speed of the impulses will determine the configuration of the P waves. (see Fig. 3.3)

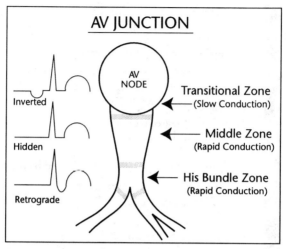

*Fig. 3-3. P wave Configurations.*

**Ventricular escape** rhythms have wide and bizarre shaped QRS complexes. Since these complexes originate from the ventricles they will appear similar to PVCs. A ventricular escape rhythm is not multiple PVCs! Ventricular escape occurs when impulses from all other higher pacemakers are absent or blocked. Ventricular escape then becomes the only mechanism from which the heart can generate pacing impulses. Treatment for ventricular escape rhythm is focused on increasing the heart rate, whereas treatment for PVCs is directed toward reducing the irritable focus with antiarrhythmic medications.

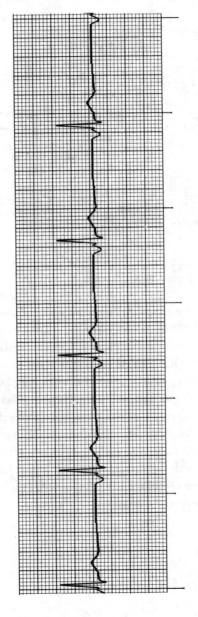

**JUNCTIONAL ESCAPE RHYTHM**

## CRITERIA

*Junctional Escape Rhythm* occurs when the SA node fails to fire or when impulses are blocked at the level of the AV node. The AV junction will usually take over as the pacemaker within 1 to 1.5 seconds of not receiving an impulse from the SA node. *Junctional escape rhythms* may be caused by ischemia or injury involving the SA node, sick sinus syndrome or digitalis toxicity.

*QRS Rate* 40 to 60 per minute.

*Rhythm* Regular.

*Atrial Activity* Inverted or absent P waves.

*QRS Width* 0.04 to 0.12 seconds.

*P to QRS Relationship* 1:1 relationship if P waves are present. P-R interval will be less than 0.12 seconds. P waves may be hidden within the QRS or appear after the QRS complexes. See Fig. 3-3.

*Treatment* If a slow ventricular rate is causing inadequate cardiac output, treatment will be directed toward increasing the rate with medication such as atropine or the application of a pacemaker. Close observation is advised.

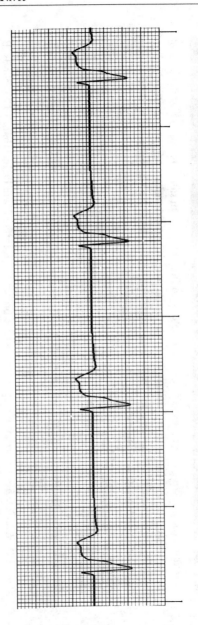

VENTRICULAR ESCAPE RHYTHM

## CRITERIA

*Ventricular Escape Rhythm*, also called idioventricular or agonal rhythm, is a safety mechanism by which the Purkinje fibers or ventricular myocardium initiate pacing impulses. This occurs when all of the impulses from the SA node or AV junction are absent or blocked. Ventricular escape is an ominous rhythm that may degenerate into asystole without rapid intervention.

*QRS Rate* Less than 40 per minute.

*Rhythm* Regular.

*Atrial Activity* Usually none. Occasional, infrequent P waves may appear throughout the rhythm.

*QRS Width* Greater than 0.12 seconds.

*P to QRS Relationship* None.

*Treatment* Treatment is directed toward increasing the ventricular rate. This rhythm may or may not respond to atropine or other medications and will usually require the application of a pacemaker.

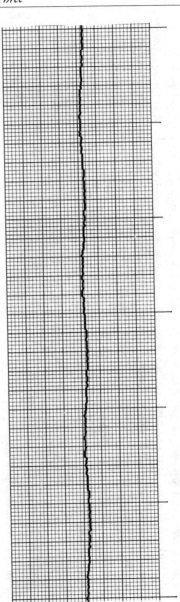

ASYSTOLE

## CRITERIA

*Asystole* indicates the absence of any pacemaker impulses. Subsequently, there is no depolarization or contraction of the ventricles. Loss of consciousness will occur within seconds and death within minutes if a viable rhythm cannot be restored. *Asystole* is caused by severe heart disease and may be precipitated by hypoxia, electrolyte imbalances, adverse medication reactions, or a myocardial infarction. It is often the terminal rhythm following unsuccessful resuscitation attempts.

*QRS Rate* None.

*Rhythm* None.

*Atrial Activity* None. Note: P waves or electronic pacemaker spikes may be seen without any QRS complexes.

*QRS Width* No QRS complexes present.

*P to QRS Relationship* None.

*Treatment* Treatment is directed toward restoration of electrical activity and may include drugs such as Epinephrine or Atropine. CPR should be implemented until a rhythm is restored or efforts are terminated. Note: improperly attached leads may show a straight line on the monitor—always check your patient and leads before initiating any treatment.

## Scenarios

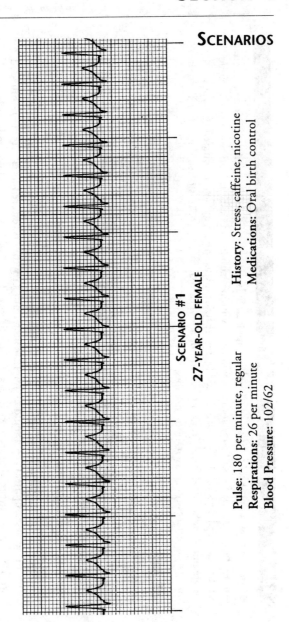

### Scenario #1
### 27-year-old female

**Pulse:** 180 per minute, regular
**Respirations:** 26 per minute
**Blood Pressure:** 102/62

**History:** Stress, caffeine, nicotine
**Medications:** Oral birth control

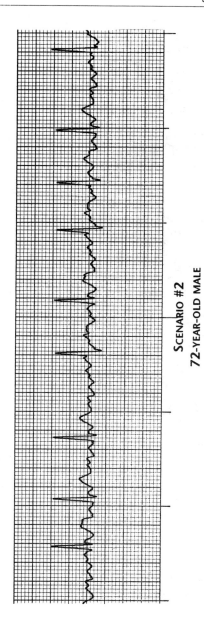

## SCENARIO #2
### 72-YEAR-OLD MALE

**Pulse:** 90 per minute, irregular
**Respirations:** 20 per minute
**Blood Pressure:** 160/84

**History:** Hernia, MI three years ago
**Medications:** Lasix, digoxin

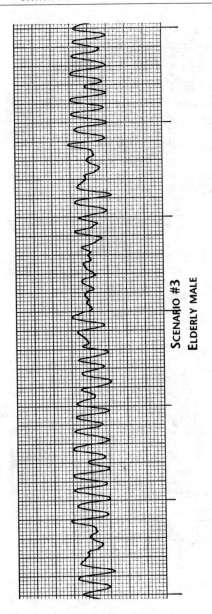

**Scenario #3**
**Elderly Male**

**Pulse:** No pulse
**Respirations:** Assisted
**Blood Pressure:** None

**History:** Unknown
**Medications:** Unknown

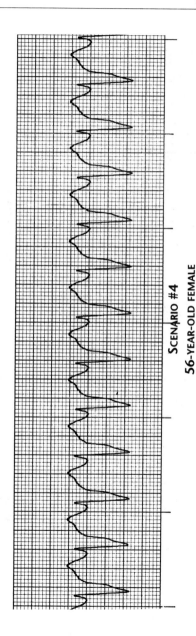

## SCENARIO #4
### 56-YEAR-OLD FEMALE

**Pulse:** 120, regular
**Respirations:** 14 via ventilator
**Blood Pressure:** 96/40

**History:** Severe GI bleeding
**Medications:** Cimetidine, vasopressin

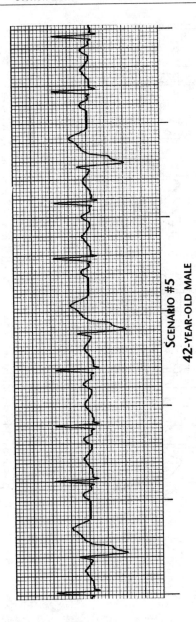

SCENARIO #5
42-YEAR-OLD MALE

Pulse: 98, irregular
Respirations: 24, wheezes
Blood Pressure: 136/80

History: asthma, acute substernal chest pain
Medications: Ventolin inhaler

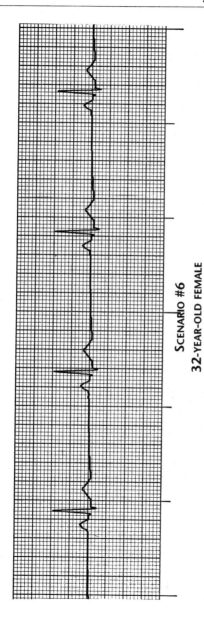

**SCENARIO #6**
**32-YEAR-OLD FEMALE**

**Pulse:** 40, regular
**Respirations:** 6 and assisted
**Blood Pressure:** 100/40

**History:** Suspected barbiturate overdose
**Medications:** Unknown

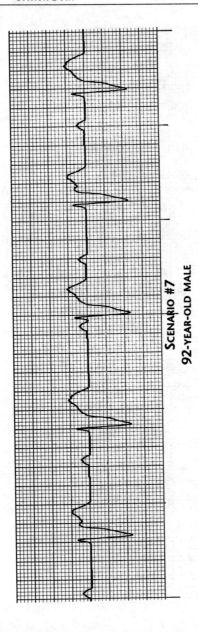

SCENARIO #7
92-YEAR-OLD MALE

Pulse: 50, regular
Respirations: 18 per minute
Blood Pressure: 188/82

History: Stroke, two previous MIs semi-conscious
Medications: Inderal, Zantac

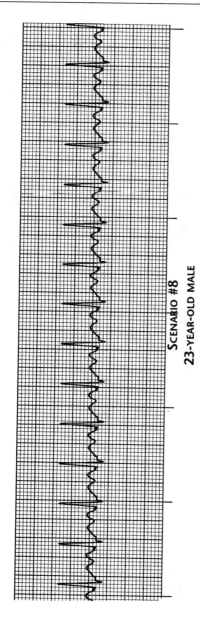

## SCENARIO #8
### 23-YEAR-OLD MALE

Pulse: 150, regular
Respirations: 26 per minute
Blood Pressure: 112/78

History: Bleeding laceration
Medications: None

# SECTION 5

## SELF-TEST

1. The branch of the autonomic nervous system that slows the heart rate is the:
   - a. sympathetic
   - b. parasympathetic
   - c. inotropic
   - d. chronotropic

2. The P wave represents the firing of the:
   - a. SA node
   - b. AV node
   - c. Purkinje fibers
   - d. ventricular myocardium

3. The QRS complex represents:
   - a. atrial depolarization
   - b. normal delay in the AV node
   - c. ventricular depolarization
   - d. ventricular repolarization

4. The T wave represents:
   - a. atrial repolarization
   - b. atrial depolarization
   - c. ventricular repolarization
   - d. ventricular depolarization

5. Which heart rate is considered bradycardia?
   - a. less than 150 per minute
   - b. less than 100 per minute
   - c. less than 80 per minute
   - d. less than 60 per minute

6. Which heart rate is typical of atrial tachycardia?

    a. 100 to 150 per minute

    b. 160 to 250 per minute

    c. 200 to 350 per minute

    d. greater than 350 per minute

7. What is the normal P-R interval?

    a. 0.12 to 0.20 seconds

    b. 0.04 to 0.12 seconds

    c. 0.04 to 0.20 seconds

    d. greater than 0.20 seconds

8. What is the normal QRS width?

    a. 0.12 to 0.20 seconds

    b. 0.04 to 0.12 seconds

    c. 0.04 to 0.20 seconds

    d. greater than 0.20 seconds

9. Indicators of the adequacy of the cardiac output include:

    a. blood pressure

    b. mental status

    c. urine output

    d. pulse

    e. all of the above

10. One small box on the ECG graph paper equals:

    a. 0.20 seconds

    b. 0.04 seconds

    c. one second

    d. three seconds

11. One large box on the ECG graph paper equals:

    a. 0.20 seconds

    b. 0.04 seconds

    c. one seconds

    d. three seconds

12. Using the "3 to 5 rule," a sinus rhythm with four large boxes between each R-R interval would be:

    a. sinus tachycardia
    b. sinus bradycardia
    c. sinus arrest
    d. normal sinus rhythm

13. A normal sinus rhythm suddenly changes to an atrial tachycardia. This is called:

    a. abrupt transition
    b. paroxysmal
    c. autonomic tachycardia
    d. chronotropic tachycardia

14. The ventricles are not being completely filled with blood from the atria when:

    a. the QRS complex is absent
    b. the R-R interval is irregular
    c. the T wave is absent
    d. the P wave is absent

15. Junctional complexes can be identified by:

    a. inverted P waves
    b. hidden P waves
    c. P waves following the QRS
    d. all of the above

16. The term for PVCs with more than one configuration within the same ECG is called:

    a. multifocal
    b. unifocal
    c. bigeminy
    d. trigeminy

17. Ventricular tachycardia is considered:

    a. normal in athletes and children
    b. to be well tolerated
    c. a lethal dysrhythmia
    d. always benign

18. Ideally, the initial treatment for V-fib is:
    a. epinephrine
    b. atropine
    c. defibrillation
    d. synchronized cardioversion

19. Ventricular dysrhythmias have in common:
    a. retrograde P waves
    b. inverted P waves
    c. wide QRS complexes
    d. normal P-R intervals

20. Which two AV blocks have variable P-R intervals? (Circle all that apply)
    a. first-degree
    b. second-degree type I
    c. second-degree type II
    d. third-degree

21. AV blocks typically have:
    a. a paroxysmal onset
    b. rapid ventricular rates
    c. slow ventricular rates
    d. no P waves

## TRUE OR FALSE

22. V-tach always generates a palpable pulse.

23. The most effective treatment for third-degree block is usually a pacemaker.

24. First-degree block indicates a delay in conduction through the AV node.

25. Digitalis toxicity can produce fast or slow dysrhythmias.

26. Escape rhythms stem from an irritable focus.

27. Fibrillatory waves may be seen in both atrial and ventricular dysrhythmias.

28. If a patient has a pulse, it will be felt during the QRS complex.

29. The ECG provides information about the mechanical activity of the heart.

30. Sinus arrhythmia may be related to breathing.

31. A loose lead can mimic V-fib or asystole.

32. In atrial fibrillation, the R-R intervals are usually irregular.

## SELF-TEST ANSWERS

| | | |
|---|---|---|
| 1. b | 12. d | 23. true |
| 2. a | 13. b | 24. true |
| 3. c | 14. d | 25. true |
| 4. c | 15. d | 26. false |
| 5. d | 16. a | 27. true |
| 6. b | 17. c | 28. true |
| 7. a | 18. c | 29. false |
| 8. b | 19. c | 30. true |
| 9. e | 20. b & d | 31. true |
| 10. b | 21. c | 32. true |
| 11. a | 22. false | |